PALEO DIET COOKBOOK

The Ultimate Guide To Delicious Paleo Recipes For Every Meal, Including Breakfast, Lunch, Dinner, Snack, Dessert, Refreshing Beverages And Occasion

Charlotte Harry

Table of Contents

CHAPTER ONE

INTRODUCTION TO THE PALEO DIET

What Is The Paleo Diet?

The Paleo diet, often referred to as the Paleolithic diet or caveman diet, is a nutritional plan designed to mimic the eating habits of our ancient ancestors from the Paleolithic era, which spanned over 2.5 million years ago. The fundamental concept of the Paleo diet is to consume foods that would have been available to humans before the development of agriculture and the advent of processed foods. This means focusing on a diet rich in whole, unprocessed foods, similar to what our hunter-gatherer ancestors would have eaten.

At the heart of the Paleo diet are lean meats, fish, fruits, vegetables, nuts, and seeds. These foods are believed to align more closely with the natural dietary patterns of early humans, potentially offering a range of health benefits. Lean meats and fish provide high-quality protein and essential fatty acids, while fruits and vegetables supply vital vitamins, minerals, and antioxidants. Nuts and seeds contribute healthy fats and additional nutrients, promoting overall wellness.

The Paleo diet excludes foods that became part of the human diet after the advent of agriculture. This includes dairy products, legumes, grains, and processed foods. The rationale behind this exclusion is that our bodies may not have fully adapted to these foods, and their consumption could contribute to various health issues. Dairy products, for example, are often avoided because many people are lactose intolerant or have difficulty digesting lactose, the sugar found in milk. Legumes and grains are excluded due to their content of antinutrients, which are substances that can interfere with the absorption of essential nutrients and may cause digestive issues in some individuals.

Processed foods are also eliminated in the Paleo diet because they often contain added sugars, unhealthy fats, and artificial additives, which can negatively impact health. By avoiding these foods, the Paleo diet aims to reduce the risk of chronic diseases, such as obesity, diabetes, heart disease, and certain types of cancer.

Adherents of the Paleo diet believe that by eating in a way that closely resembles the dietary patterns of our Paleolithic ancestors, they can achieve optimal health and well-being. This approach emphasizes the consumption of nutrient-dense, natural foods that support overall health and vitality. The diet encourages individuals to pay close attention to the quality of their food, choosing organic, grass-fed, and wild-caught options whenever possible to maximize the nutritional benefits.

The Paleo diet advocates for a return to the dietary habits of our ancient ancestors, focusing on whole, unprocessed foods while excluding modern agricultural products and processed foods. This approach aims to promote optimal health by aligning our eating patterns with those that our bodies are naturally adapted to.

History And Evolution Of The Paleo Diet

The Paleo diet, rooted in the dietary habits of our ancient hunter-gatherer ancestors, gained widespread attention in the early 2000s. This dietary approach emerged from the observation that early humans, who thrived on a diet of wild plants and animals, were free from many of the chronic diseases prevalent today, such as obesity, diabetes, and heart disease. The rationale behind the Paleo diet is that our bodies are genetically adapted to the foods available in the Paleolithic era, and thus, by reverting to this ancient way of eating, modern individuals can achieve optimal health.

The diet emphasizes whole, unprocessed foods that would have been available to our prehistoric ancestors. This includes lean meats, fish, fruits, vegetables, nuts, and seeds. It excludes foods that became common with the advent of agriculture and industrial food processing, such as grains, legumes, dairy products, refined sugars, and processed oils. The premise is that these latter foods are at odds with our genetic makeup, contributing to the rise of chronic health issues.

Over time, the Paleo diet has evolved and diversified. Different variations and adaptations have emerged, each with its own interpretation of what constitutes an ideal Paleo diet. Some versions strictly adhere to the original concept, avoiding all foods that were not available to Paleolithic humans. Others adopt a more flexible approach, allowing for some modern foods that are considered to be healthy and minimally processed. For example, some proponents include certain dairy products, such as grass-fed butter or fermented yogurt, arguing that these foods can offer health benefits while still being relatively natural and unprocessed.

Despite these variations, the core principle of the Paleo diet remains consistent: to consume foods that are as close as possible to what early humans ate. This means prioritizing nutrient-dense, whole foods and avoiding highly processed items. Advocates of the diet argue that this approach not only supports physical health but also aligns with our evolutionary biology, helping to prevent and mitigate chronic diseases.

The popularity of the Paleo diet has led to extensive research and discussion within the health and nutrition communities. Studies have explored its potential benefits, including weight loss, improved metabolic health, and reduced inflammation. Critics, however, point out that there is no one-size-fits-all approach to diet and that individual nutritional needs can vary widely.

Benefits Of The Paleo Diet

The Paleo diet, often referred to as the "caveman diet," is praised by its proponents for offering numerous health benefits rooted in the consumption of whole, nutrient-dense foods. At the heart of the Paleo philosophy is the belief that by eating in a manner similar to our prehistoric ancestors, we can improve our overall health and well-being. This approach emphasizes the intake of unprocessed foods that are rich in vitamins, minerals, and antioxidants, which play a crucial role in supporting the immune system, reducing inflammation, and boosting energy levels.

One of the primary benefits of the Paleo diet is its focus on nutrient-dense foods. These foods, which include fruits, vegetables, lean meats, fish, nuts, and seeds, provide a rich source of essential nutrients that are vital for maintaining optimal health. For instance, fruits and vegetables are loaded with vitamins and minerals, such as vitamin C, potassium, and magnesium, which are essential for various bodily functions. The high antioxidant content in these foods helps combat oxidative stress and inflammation, potentially reducing the risk of chronic diseases.

In addition to promoting nutrient-dense foods, the Paleo diet also eliminates processed foods and refined sugars. Processed foods often contain unhealthy additives, preservatives, and trans fats, which have been linked to a host of health problems, including obesity, diabetes, and heart disease. By cutting out these foods, individuals following the Paleo diet may experience significant health improvements. For example, the elimination of refined sugars can lead to better blood sugar control, reducing the risk of developing type 2 diabetes.

Furthermore, avoiding processed foods can contribute to weight loss and improved cardiovascular health, as these foods are typically high in unhealthy fats and empty calories.

Another key aspect of the Paleo diet is its emphasis on protein intake. Protein is essential for building and maintaining muscle mass, which is crucial for overall physical health and metabolic function. Lean meats, fish, and eggs are staple sources of protein in the Paleo diet, providing the necessary amino acids required for muscle repair and growth. Additionally, a high-protein diet can enhance satiety, helping individuals feel fuller for longer periods and potentially reducing overall calorie intake, which can support weight loss efforts.

Overall, the Paleo diet's focus on whole, nutrient-dense foods, the elimination of processed and refined foods, and its high protein content contribute to its potential health benefits. These benefits include improved nutrition, enhanced immune function, reduced inflammation, better weight management, improved blood sugar control, and cardiovascular health. While individual results may vary, many find that adopting the Paleo lifestyle leads to a healthier, more balanced approach to eating.

Paleo Diet Myths And Misconceptions

Despite its rising popularity, the Paleo diet is often surrounded by myths and misconceptions that can cloud its true nature and benefits. A common myth is that the Paleo diet is excessively restrictive and challenging to follow. While it does involve the elimination of certain food groups such as grains, legumes, and dairy, it still offers a wide array of delicious and nutritious foods. Adherents can enjoy a variety of meats, fish, fruits, vegetables, nuts, and seeds. This diversity ensures that meals can be flavorful and satisfying, making the diet more manageable than some might believe.

Another prevalent misconception is that the Paleo diet is purely meat-based. This myth likely stems from the diet's emphasis on consuming animal products as part of a return to the eating patterns of our hunter-gatherer ancestors. However, the Paleo diet actually promotes a balanced intake of both animal and plant-based foods. It encourages the consumption of ample fruits and vegetables, which provide essential vitamins, minerals, and fiber. This balance helps ensure that the diet is not only varied but also nutritionally complete, countering the misconception that it is overly reliant on meat.

Critics of the Paleo diet often argue that it lacks scientific evidence to support its health claims. While it is true that long-term, large-scale studies specifically on the Paleo diet are limited, there is a substantial body of research highlighting the benefits of eating whole, unprocessed foods, which is a core principle of the diet. Studies have shown that diets rich in whole foods can help reduce the risk of chronic diseases such as heart disease, diabetes, and obesity. Furthermore, the elimination of processed foods and refined sugars, which are linked to numerous health issues, aligns with broader nutritional advice for maintaining a healthy lifestyle.

One additional myth is that the Paleo diet is a one-size-fits-all approach. In reality, it can be adapted to individual preferences and needs. For instance, those who are more active may require more carbohydrates, which can be obtained from Paleo-friendly sources like sweet potatoes and fruits. The flexibility within the framework of the Paleo diet allows for personalization, making it suitable for a wide range of individuals with different health goals and dietary needs.

Getting Started With The Paleo Diet

Starting the Paleo diet can initially seem overwhelming, but with a systematic approach, it becomes manageable and rewarding. The first step is to gradually eliminate processed foods, refined sugars, grains, legumes, and dairy products from your diet. Instead of making these changes abruptly, ease into them by slowly reducing the intake of these items. This gradual transition can help your body adjust without feeling deprived or overwhelmed.

Focus on incorporating more whole foods into your meals. Lean meats, fish, fruits, vegetables, nuts, and seeds should become staples in your diet. These foods are nutrient-dense and align with the principles of the Paleo diet, which emphasizes eating as our ancestors did. When selecting meats, opt for grass-fed or pasture-raised options, as these are typically higher in beneficial nutrients.

Similarly, choose wild-caught fish when possible.

Meal planning and preparation are key to success on the Paleo diet. Dedicate time each week to plan your meals and prepare food in advance. This not only saves time but also ensures that you always have Paleo-friendly options available, reducing the temptation to revert to non-Paleo foods. Batch cooking can be particularly useful; prepare large quantities of meals and store them for the week ahead.

Hydration is another crucial aspect. Drink plenty of water throughout the day to support your body's functions and overall health. Listening to your body is equally important; it will signal if certain foods do not agree with you or if you need more of a particular nutrient. Be attentive to these signals and adjust your food choices accordingly.

Seeking support from others who follow the Paleo diet can provide valuable motivation and tips. Online communities, social media groups, and local meetups can offer a wealth of knowledge and encouragement. Engaging with others on the same journey can make the transition smoother and more enjoyable.

The overarching goal of the Paleo diet is to make sustainable changes that promote long-term health and well-being. This is not about short-term fixes or extreme restrictions but about adopting a way of eating that supports your body naturally. By embracing the principles of the Paleo diet, you can enjoy a nutritious and satisfying way of eating that aligns with our ancestral roots. This approach not only benefits your physical health but also contributes to overall wellness, fostering a balanced and fulfilling lifestyle.

Ultimately, the Paleo diet is about making thoughtful choices that enhance your quality of life. With patience and persistence, these changes will become second nature, leading to lasting health benefits and a deeper connection to natural, wholesome foods.

CHAPTER TWO

PALEO DIET BASICS

Approved Foods And Ingredients

When starting the Paleo diet, understanding the spectrum of approved foods is crucial. Rooted in the premise of emulating ancestral eating habits from the Paleolithic era, this dietary approach champions whole, unprocessed foods for optimal health and vitality.

Central to the Paleo diet are various categories of approved foods:

Meat and Poultry: Key selections encompass beef, pork, chicken, turkey, and lamb. Opting for grass-fed or pasture-raised varieties enhances nutritional benefits, aligning closely with the diet's principles.

Fish and Seafood: Embracing the bounty of the sea, Paleo enthusiasts favor wild-caught fish such as salmon, tuna, and cod. Additionally, shellfish like shrimp and crab are celebrated for their nutrient density and compatibility with the diet.

Eggs: A cornerstone of Paleo-friendly protein sources, free-range or organic eggs are preferred for their superior nutritional profile, contributing to a balanced diet foundation.

Vegetables: Virtually all vegetables find a place within the Paleo spectrum, with a nod toward nutrient-dense options like leafy greens, cruciferous vegetables (e.g., broccoli, cauliflower), and root vegetables such as carrots and sweet potatoes. These vegetables offer essential vitamins, minerals, and fiber crucial for overall well-being.

Fruits: Paleo-friendly fruits include berries, apples, bananas, and oranges. While these fruits provide valuable nutrients, individuals mindful of sugar intake for weight management may moderate consumption accordingly.

Nuts and Seeds: Almonds, walnuts, sunflower seeds, and chia seeds are revered for their nutritional benefits in Paleo circles. Rich in healthy fats, protein, and fiber, they serve as versatile additions to meals or satisfying snacks.

Healthy Fats: Integral to cooking and flavoring in Paleo cuisine, olive oil, coconut oil, avocado, and ghee (clarified butter) are lauded for their beneficial fats and distinctive tastes, enhancing both culinary creations and overall dietary balance.

Herbs and Spices: Offering culinary flair without excess calories, herbs and spices form an essential part of the Paleo diet. From basil and thyme to turmeric and cinnamon, these ingredients elevate dishes while contributing antioxidants and other health-promoting compounds.

Foods To Avoid

Understanding what to avoid is crucial on the Paleo diet, which centers around consuming foods that our early ancestors would have eaten. This approach excludes modern processed foods, grains, legumes, dairy, refined sugars, and certain vegetable oils due to their potential health impacts.

Processed Foods: The Paleo diet steers clear of processed foods, which are laden with artificial additives, preservatives, and chemicals. These include pre-packaged snacks, frozen meals, and fast food. By eliminating these, adherents aim to return to whole, natural foods that support optimal health and well-being.

Grains: Wheat, rice, oats, barley, and other grains are omitted from the Paleo diet. The rationale behind this exclusion is that grains were not part of our early ancestors' diet. Instead, the focus is on nutrient-dense alternatives like vegetables, fruits, and nuts.

Legumes: Legumes such as beans, lentils, chickpeas, and peanuts are avoided due to their content of anti-nutrients such as lectins and phytates. These compounds can interfere with nutrient absorption in the gut, which contrasts with the Paleo philosophy of promoting efficient digestion and nutrient utilization.

Dairy: Despite its widespread consumption today, dairy products like milk, cheese, and yogurt are not included in the Paleo diet. This exclusion is based on the belief that early humans did not consume dairy beyond infancy and that lactose intolerance among adults suggests it may not be universally well-tolerated.

Refined Sugars: White sugar, brown sugar, and high-fructose corn syrup are restricted on the Paleo diet due to their adverse effects on blood sugar levels and overall health. Instead, natural sweeteners like honey or maple syrup may be used sparingly to add sweetness to dishes without the drawbacks associated with refined sugars.

Vegetable Oils: Oils derived from vegetables such as canola, soybean, and corn oil are avoided because of their high omega-6 fatty acid content. Excessive consumption of these oils has been linked to inflammation, which contradicts the anti-inflammatory principles emphasized in the Paleo diet. Instead, oils like olive oil or coconut oil, which are richer in beneficial fats, are preferred.

Understanding Macros: Protein, Carbs, And Fats

In the realm of the Paleo diet, achieving a balanced intake of macronutrients—protein, carbohydrates, and fats—is fundamental for sustaining optimal health and energy levels.

Protein: Protein serves as a cornerstone for building and repairing tissues within the body. In the context of the Paleo diet, protein sources primarily derive from animal products such as meat, fish, and eggs. These sources are rich in essential amino acids, which are crucial for maintaining muscle mass, supporting immune function, and facilitating enzymatic processes. The Paleo approach encourages including a protein source in every meal to promote satiety and muscle recovery. Whether it's a serving of grilled chicken, a portion of wild-caught salmon, or eggs prepared in various forms, prioritizing protein intake ensures that the body receives ample support for its structural and functional needs.

Carbohydrates: Carbohydrates serve as the primary fuel source for the body, powering daily activities and maintaining metabolic functions. In contrast to conventional diets that often rely on grains and refined sugars, the Paleo diet emphasizes carbohydrates sourced from nutrient-dense, fiber-rich vegetables and fruits. Examples include sweet potatoes, squash, broccoli, and leafy greens. These choices not only provide carbohydrates but also deliver essential vitamins, minerals, and dietary fiber. By focusing on these natural, unprocessed sources, adherents of the Paleo diet aim to stabilize blood sugar levels, enhance digestion, and promote sustained energy throughout the day. This approach not only supports overall health but also aligns with the diet's philosophy of consuming foods that our ancestors would have had access to during the Paleolithic era.

Fats: Healthy fats play a critical role in promoting brain health, facilitating hormone production, and providing a concentrated source of energy. Within the Paleo framework, approved fat sources include avocados, nuts, seeds, and oils like olive and coconut oil. These fats are celebrated for their nutrient density and beneficial fatty acid profiles, such as omega-3s and monounsaturated fats. Incorporating these fats into meals not only enhances flavor and texture but also contributes to feelings of fullness and satisfaction. Whether drizzling olive oil over a salad, enjoying a handful of almonds as a snack, or adding avocado to a meal, integrating these healthy fats ensures that the body receives essential nutrients while supporting overall well-being.

Stocking your pantry with essentials for a Paleo diet is crucial for maintaining a healthy and satisfying meal plan. By ensuring you have these key items on hand, you can easily adhere to Paleo guidelines while preparing delicious meals and snacks.

First and foremost, coconut oil and olive oil are indispensable. Coconut oil is ideal for cooking at higher temperatures, thanks to its stable composition, while olive oil is perfect for dressings and lower-heat cooking, providing healthy fats essential to the diet.

When it comes to baking and creating Paleo-friendly treats, having coconut flour and almond flour is essential. These flours are gluten-free alternatives that impart a delicious texture and flavor to various recipes, from bread to cookies.

Nuts and seeds are versatile staples that offer protein and healthy fats. Keep a variety like almonds, walnuts, and chia seeds on hand for snacking or incorporating into salads and other dishes.

Canned fish, such as salmon and tuna, are convenient sources of protein rich in omega-3 fatty acids. They are perfect for quick meals like salads or as a protein component in larger dishes.

Spices and herbs are vital for adding flavor without relying on processed ingredients. A well-stocked pantry should include a variety of these, such as basil, oregano, and turmeric, ensuring your meals are both tasty and nutritious.

Broth and bone broth are excellent bases for soups and stews, offering not only flavor but also important nutrients like collagen and minerals. They provide a hearty foundation for Paleo-friendly meals.

In moderation, dried fruits like raisins and apricots can be used to add natural sweetness to dishes or enjoyed as snacks. They provide a burst of flavor and a touch of sweetness without added sugars or artificial ingredients.

Meal Planning And Prepping

Meal planning and prepping are essential components of a successful Paleo diet regimen, ensuring you stay on track with your nutritional goals and simplify your daily routines. By strategizing your meals in advance and preparing them efficiently, you can optimize your time and maintain consistency in your dietary choices.

Firstly, effective meal planning begins with deciding your weekly meals based on Paleo-approved foods and essential pantry items. This proactive approach not only streamlines your grocery shopping but also helps you avoid impulse purchases of non-compliant foods. Creating a detailed shopping list ensures you have everything you need, minimizing last-minute stress and ensuring you're well-prepared for the week ahead.

Once you have your ingredients, dedicating a day to meal preparation can significantly lighten your weekday workload. Use this time to chop vegetables, marinate meats, and assemble meals that can be easily cooked during the week. By prepping ingredients ahead of time, you can reduce cooking time on busy days, making it more convenient to stick to your dietary plan.

Cooking in batches is another valuable strategy. Prepare large quantities of meals such as soups, stews, and casseroles that can be stored in the refrigerator or freezer. This approach not only saves time but also ensures you have nutritious options readily available, especially when time is tight.

For snacking, keep Paleo-friendly options like nuts, seeds, and fruits within reach. Portion them into convenient containers or snack packs so you can grab them on the go without compromising your dietary goals. This helps curb cravings and provides sustained energy throughout the day.

Organization plays a pivotal role in maintaining your Paleo lifestyle. Use clear containers to store prepped meals and snacks, and label them with contents and dates for easy identification. This keeps your fridge and pantry tidy and ensures that you always know what's available for meals or snacks.

CHAPTER THREE

BREAKFAST RECIPES

Paleo Pancakes And Waffle

Embracing the Paleo diet isn't just about following a set of rules; it's about reimagining beloved comfort foods with ingredients that not only adhere to Paleo guidelines but also enhance nutritional value. A prime example of this culinary creativity lies in Paleo pancakes and waffles, where traditional wheat flour gives way to nutrient-dense alternatives like almond flour, coconut flour, or a blend of both. These substitutes not only sidestep grains but also enrich these breakfast classics with increased protein and healthy fats, making them a wholesome choice for Paleo enthusiasts.

Paleo pancake and waffle recipes typically revolve around a base of almond flour, coconut flour, or a combination thereof. Almond flour, derived from finely ground almonds, brings a subtly sweet flavor and a moist texture, while coconut flour, made from dried coconut meat, adds a lightness and a hint of natural sweetness. Combining these flours balances their individual characteristics, resulting in a satisfying texture that closely mimics traditional pancakes and waffles.

Central to many Paleo recipes are eggs, which act as a binding agent and contribute to the overall structure of pancakes and waffles. Eggs also provide a significant protein boost, essential for a balanced Paleo meal. Coconut milk often replaces traditional dairy, adding a creamy richness that complements the flavors of almond and coconut flours. This substitution not only aligns with Paleo principles but also caters to those avoiding lactose or seeking a dairy-free option.

For natural sweetness, Paleo pancake and waffle recipes commonly incorporate fruits such as berries or mashed bananas. These fruits not only infuse a delightful flavor but also contribute essential vitamins, minerals, and dietary fiber. Their natural sugars offer a healthier alternative to refined sugars, aligning with the Paleo emphasis on whole, unprocessed foods.

The versatility of Paleo pancakes and waffles extends beyond their base ingredients. Variations abound, allowing for customization according to personal preferences and dietary needs. Some recipes may include additional ingredients like vanilla extract for flavor depth, cinnamon for warmth, or even a touch of honey or maple syrup for a touch of sweetness, keeping within moderation guidelines.

In essence, Paleo pancakes and waffles exemplify the innovative spirit of the Paleo diet, transforming familiar breakfast staples into nourishing meals that support overall health and wellness. By embracing nutrient-dense alternatives and natural ingredients, these recipes not only satisfy cravings but also promote a balanced approach to eating that resonates with Paleo principles. Whether enjoyed plain or adorned with fresh fruit and a drizzle of natural sweeteners, Paleo pancakes and waffles offer a delicious reminder that eating well can be both satisfying and nutritious.

Egg-Based Breakfasts

In the realm of Paleo cuisine, eggs reign supreme as a cornerstone ingredient, valued not only for their robust protein profile but also for their adaptability across a spectrum of dishes. This section delves into the art of crafting wholesome breakfasts centered around eggs, showcasing their versatility and nutritional prowess within the Paleo framework.

Eggs serve as a foundational element in countless Paleo recipes, celebrated for their ability to provide sustained energy and satiety. Whether scrambled, transformed into a fluffy omelet, or baked into a hearty frittata, their culinary potential knows no bounds. Each preparation method offers a unique texture and flavor profile, making eggs an ideal canvas for creative Paleo breakfast creations.

Scrambled eggs, a timeless favorite, epitomize simplicity and quick preparation without sacrificing nutritional density. Enhanced with vibrant vegetables such as spinach, bell peppers, and earthy mushrooms, these scrambled eggs elevate breakfast to a nutrient-packed affair. The addition of these vegetables not only boosts flavor but also enriches the dish with essential vitamins, minerals, and dietary fiber, essential components of a balanced Paleo meal.

Omelets, another stalwart in the Paleo breakfast repertoire, allow for endless customization. Folded around a medley of sautéed vegetables and perhaps a hint of

Paleo-friendly cheese or herbs, omelets showcase the marriage of flavors and textures in a single satisfying dish. The richness of eggs complements the freshness of ingredients like diced tomatoes, onions, and kale, offering a robust start to the day.

Frittatas, a more substantial option, combine the goodness of eggs with an array of ingredients baked to perfection. Packed with protein and nutrients, frittatas effortlessly accommodate Paleo principles with ingredients such as diced sweet potatoes, bacon, and even leftover roasted vegetables from previous meals. This make-ahead dish not only simplifies mornings but also ensures a hearty, nutrient-dense breakfast option for busy Paleo enthusiasts.

For those seeking variety, eggs can be paired with Paleo staples like creamy avocado slices, zesty salsa, or leftover roasted vegetables. These additions not only enhance the flavor but also contribute additional nutrients and healthy fats, aligning perfectly with the Paleo philosophy of whole, unprocessed foods.

In essence, this section celebrates eggs as a nutritional powerhouse within the Paleo diet, offering a range of breakfast ideas that cater to both taste and health. Whether enjoyed simply scrambled, elegantly folded into an omelet, or baked into a satisfying frittata, eggs provide a versatile foundation for crafting nutrient-packed Paleo breakfasts that nourish and satisfy.

Smoothies And Shakes

Smoothies and shakes are a cornerstone of the Paleo diet, offering a convenient and nutrient-dense way to kickstart your day or refuel after a workout. These beverages epitomize the Paleo philosophy by focusing on natural, whole-food ingredients that provide sustained energy and promote overall wellness.

At the heart of Paleo-friendly smoothies are fresh, wholesome components that blend seamlessly into a delicious concoction. Leafy greens such as kale or spinach form a nutritional base, packing in essential vitamins, minerals, and fiber. These greens not only contribute to the vibrant color of the smoothie but also offer a refreshing earthy taste that complements the sweetness of fruits.

Speaking of fruits, Paleo smoothies often feature a variety of nature's candies: berries bursting with antioxidants, tropical delights like mango, or the tangy sweetness of pineapple. These fruits not only enhance flavor but also provide natural sugars that are balanced by the fiber content, supporting stable blood sugar levels—a key aspect of the Paleo approach.

To add creaminess and healthy fats, many Paleo enthusiasts turn to alternatives like coconut milk or avocado. These ingredients not only lend a silky texture to the smoothie but also offer a rich source of medium-chain triglycerides (MCTs) and essential fatty acids, promoting satiety and supporting brain health.

Protein is another essential component of Paleo smoothies, often sourced from ingredients like almond butter or collagen powder. These additions not only boost the protein content but also contribute to muscle repair and recovery—a perfect complement for those leading an active lifestyle.

What makes Paleo smoothies truly versatile is their adaptability to personal taste preferences and dietary needs. Whether you prefer a tropical twist with coconut and pineapple or a berry blast with antioxidant-rich berries, the combinations are endless. This customization ensures that each smoothie is not only nutritious but also enjoyable, making it easier to stick to a Paleo lifestyle.

Beyond their nutritional benefits, Paleo smoothies and shakes offer practicality in a busy world. They can be prepared quickly, making them ideal for hectic mornings or as a post-workout refuel. By incorporating Paleo principles into these beverages, individuals can harness the power of natural ingredients to support their health goals while savoring the delicious flavors that Mother Nature provides.

Grain-Free Breakfast Bowls

Grain-free breakfast bowls are a delightful twist on traditional morning meals, eschewing oats and wheat in favor of nutrient-rich alternatives like chia seeds, flaxseed meal, and shredded coconut. These ingredients not only offer a satisfying texture but also pack a nutritional punch, delivering fiber, healthy fats, and essential nutrients that are integral to a balanced Paleo diet.

Chia seeds, known for their omega-3 fatty acids and fiber content, provide a gel-like consistency when mixed with liquid, creating a base that's both filling and nutritious. Flaxseed meal, rich in lignans and fiber, adds a nutty flavor and boosts digestive health. Meanwhile, shredded coconut contributes a natural sweetness and a dose of medium-chain triglycerides (MCTs), which are easily metabolized by the body for quick energy.

What sets grain-free breakfast bowls apart is their versatility. They serve as a blank canvas for creativity, allowing Paleo enthusiasts to customize their bowls to suit personal tastes and dietary needs. Toppings can range from crunchy nuts and seeds, which add texture and protein, to vibrant fresh fruits that provide natural sweetness and a spectrum of vitamins and antioxidants. For added richness, a drizzle of coconut milk or almond butter not only enhances flavor but also boosts the bowl's nutrient profile with healthy fats.

These bowls are not just a nutritious breakfast option but also a practical one. They cater to individuals seeking to avoid grains due to dietary restrictions or preferences, offering a satisfying alternative that doesn't compromise on taste or nutrition. By incorporating a variety of wholesome ingredients, grain-free breakfast bowls ensure that each bite is packed with flavor and goodness, supporting sustained energy levels throughout the morning.

For Paleo followers, these bowls represent more than just a meal—they embody a commitment to wholesome eating and nourishment. Whether enjoyed as a quick weekday breakfast or a leisurely weekend treat, grain-free breakfast bowls showcase the delicious possibilities of Paleo cooking, proving that healthy eating can be both enjoyable and fulfilling.

Breakfast On The Go

One of the staples of a Paleo breakfast on the go is homemade energy bars. These bars are packed with nuts, dates, and seeds, offering a satisfying blend of protein, healthy fats, and natural sweetness. They can be easily prepared in batches over the weekend and stored for the week ahead. With ingredients like almonds, cashews, dried fruits, and a touch of honey or maple syrup for sweetness, these bars are both delicious and nourishing.

For those who prefer a lighter option, chia seed pudding is a perfect choice. By mixing chia seeds with coconut milk or almond milk and a dash of vanilla extract, you create a creamy pudding that sets overnight in the refrigerator. In the morning, top it with fresh berries, sliced almonds, or a sprinkle of cinnamon for added flavor and texture. Chia seed pudding is not only rich in omega-3 fatty acids but also provides a good amount of fiber to keep you feeling full and satisfied until lunchtime.

If you're looking for a quick source of protein, hard-boiled eggs are an excellent grab-and-go option. They can be prepared ahead of time and stored in the refrigerator for up to a week. Pair them with a piece of fruit like an apple or banana for a balanced breakfast that combines protein with natural carbohydrates.

Nut butter packets are another convenient choice for Paleo eaters on the move. Single-serving packets of almond butter or cashew butter provide a portable source of healthy fats and protein. Spread them on slices of apple or celery sticks for a quick snack or pair them with a few squares of dark chocolate for a satisfying morning treat.

CHAPTER FOUR

LUNCH RECIPES

Fresh And Hearty Salads

Fresh and hearty salads play a pivotal role in the Paleo diet, renowned for their emphasis on fresh vegetables, lean proteins, and healthy fats. These salads embody a vibrant array of flavors and textures, typically featuring a base of nutrient-dense greens such as spinach, kale, or arugula. Complementing these greens are an assortment of colorful vegetables like juicy tomatoes, crisp cucumbers, sweet bell peppers, and creamy avocado slices, each contributing not only to taste but also to the salad's nutritional richness.

Proteins are a crucial component of Paleo salads, often including options such as grilled chicken breast, hard-boiled eggs, or succulent grilled shrimp. These lean sources of protein not only enhance satiety but also provide essential amino acids necessary for muscle repair and overall health. To elevate the salad's nutritional profile further, healthy fats are integrated through the inclusion of ingredients like drizzled olive oil or crunchy nuts and seeds such as almonds or pumpkin seeds. These fats not only add a satisfying crunch but also deliver vital omega-3 fatty acids and antioxidants.

Dressings in Paleo salads are intentionally kept simple and wholesome, steering clear of processed sugars and additives. Common dressing choices include a light drizzle of extra-virgin olive oil paired with tangy vinegar or fresh lemon juice, enhancing the salad's flavors without compromising its nutritional integrity. The emphasis on natural, unprocessed ingredients ensures that every component of the salad aligns with the Paleo philosophy of eating foods as close to their natural state as possible.

Beyond their nutritional benefits, Paleo salads offer versatility and creativity, allowing individuals to tailor them to personal tastes and dietary preferences. Whether as a refreshing side dish or a satisfying main course, these salads not only nourish the body but also celebrate the vibrant flavors and textures of fresh, wholesome ingredients. They serve as a testament to the Paleo diet's commitment to promoting health through nutrient-dense, whole foods that support overall well-being and vitality.

Paleo Wraps And Sandwiches

Paleo wraps and sandwiches offer a creative departure from traditional bread-based meals, adhering closely to the principles of the Paleo diet. This dietary approach emphasizes whole, unprocessed foods similar to those consumed by our ancestors during the Paleolithic era. By substituting conventional bread with innovative alternatives, Paleo enthusiasts can enjoy a diverse array of satisfying meals that align with their nutritional goals.

One popular substitute for bread in Paleo cuisine is the lettuce wrap. Utilizing large, sturdy leafy greens such as romaine or collard greens, these wraps serve as a wholesome vessel for a variety of fillings. For instance, grilled chicken, turkey, or tuna can be combined with creamy avocado or homemade Paleo mayonnaise, creating a flavorful and protein-rich meal. The crisp freshness of the lettuce provides a refreshing contrast to the savory fillings, making each bite both nutritious and delicious.

Another favored option is grain-free flatbreads crafted from ingredients like almond flour or coconut flour. These flatbreads offer a robust foundation that supports heartier fillings such as roasted vegetables, sliced turkey, and avocado. Rich in healthy fats and free from grains, they cater to those following a Paleo lifestyle while accommodating dietary preferences and restrictions. The versatility of these flatbreads allows for endless combinations, ensuring that every meal is both satisfying and nutritionally balanced.

What makes Paleo wraps and sandwiches particularly appealing is their adaptability. Whether you prefer a light, refreshing lettuce wrap on a warm summer day or a more substantial flatbread filled with savory ingredients, there's a Paleo option to suit every occasion. These alternatives not only satisfy cravings but also contribute to overall well-being by emphasizing whole foods and minimizing processed ingredients.

Beyond their culinary appeal, Paleo wraps and sandwiches support a holistic approach to health. By focusing on nutrient-dense ingredients and eliminating grains and refined sugars, they promote stable energy levels and optimal digestion. This dietary strategy reflects a commitment to eating in harmony with our evolutionary heritage, prioritizing foods that nourish the body and support long-term health.

Soups And Stews

Soups and stews play a crucial role in the Paleo diet, offering both comfort and nutritional density, especially during lunchtime. These dishes are crafted around wholesome ingredients, starting with a foundation of either homemade bone broth rich in collagen and minerals or vegetable broth for a lighter option. They serve as perfect vessels for a plethora of vegetables typical to the Paleo regimen, such as carrots, celery, and sweet potatoes. These vegetables not only enhance flavor but also provide essential vitamins and fiber crucial for a balanced diet.

Proteins featured in Paleo soups and stews are sourced from high-quality, organic sources like grass-fed beef, free-range chicken, or wild-caught fish. These proteins not only align with the Paleo philosophy but also contribute important nutrients like omega-3 fatty acids and lean proteins. The inclusion of these proteins ensures that these meals are not only filling but also supportive of overall health and well-being.

To deepen the complexity of flavors without relying on processed ingredients, Paleo soups and stews utilize natural seasonings such as garlic, fresh herbs like thyme and parsley, and a variety of spices. This approach not only enhances taste but also provides additional health benefits from the antioxidant and anti-inflammatory properties found in herbs and spices.

One of the key advantages of Paleo soups and stews is their suitability for batch cooking. By preparing large quantities at once, they offer a convenient solution for busy individuals looking to maintain a Paleo lifestyle without sacrificing time or nutrition. These dishes can be easily stored and reheated, making them ideal for quick and nutritious meals throughout the week.

Moreover, the nutrient density of Paleo soups and stews makes them a versatile choice, suitable for various dietary preferences and requirements. Whether aiming to boost protein intake, increase vegetable consumption, or simply enjoy a hearty and satisfying meal, these dishes deliver on both flavor and nutrition.

Protein-Packed Lunch Bowls

Protein-packed lunch bowls offer a delicious and nutritious way to integrate lean proteins, vegetables, and healthy fats into your daily diet. These bowls are not only satisfying but also versatile, allowing for endless combinations to suit various tastes and dietary preferences.

Imagine a lunch bowl featuring grilled salmon or chicken, generously layered over a base of cauliflower rice or a bed of mixed greens. This hearty foundation is complemented by creamy avocado slices, juicy cherry tomatoes, and a light drizzle of extra virgin olive oil or a splash of fresh lemon juice. The result is a vibrant, nutrient-rich meal that promises both flavor and health benefits.

For those opting for a poultry alternative, consider a bowl with seasoned ground turkey, sautéed until golden with spinach and mushrooms. Enhanced with a blend of aromatic herbs and spices, this savory mixture adds depth to each bite while providing ample protein and essential nutrients.

What makes these bowls particularly appealing is their adaptability. You can tailor them to fit specific dietary needs or flavor preferences effortlessly. For instance, substituting quinoa or sweet potatoes for cauliflower rice adds complex carbohydrates, enriching the meal with sustained energy. Alternatively, adding a sprinkle of seeds or nuts not only enhances texture but also boosts healthy fats and additional nutrients.

Beyond their culinary appeal, these protein-packed bowls are designed to support sustained energy levels and promote feelings of fullness. The combination of lean proteins, fiber-rich vegetables, and beneficial fats helps stabilize blood sugar levels, preventing energy crashes often associated with carb-heavy meals.

Whether you're meal-prepping for the week ahead or assembling a quick lunch on the go, these bowls provide a convenient solution without compromising on taste or nutrition. They exemplify the principles of balanced eating, offering a wholesome blend of macronutrients that nourish the body and satisfy the palate.

Light And Easy Lunches

In the realm of Paleo dining, a quick and nourishing lunch can be a lifesaver amidst busy schedules. These meals are designed to be both light on preparation time and rich in essential nutrients, catering to those seeking a satisfying midday meal without compromising on health.

One delightful option for a Paleo-friendly lunch is a refreshing tuna or chicken salad. Prepared with Paleo-approved mayonnaise or creamy avocado, these salads offer a burst of protein and healthy fats. They can be enjoyed atop a bed of crisp mixed greens for added freshness and texture, or elegantly wrapped in large lettuce leaves, providing a convenient and gluten-free alternative to traditional wraps. The combination of lean protein and leafy greens not only satisfies hunger but also fuels the body with essential vitamins and minerals.

For those preferring a warm option, a simple vegetable omelet cooked in coconut oil fits the bill perfectly. Packed with spinach, bell peppers, and savory mushrooms, this omelet offers a savory medley of flavors and a substantial dose of fiber. Coconut oil, renowned for its medium-chain triglycerides, adds healthy fats that support cognitive function and provide lasting energy throughout the afternoon. This versatile dish can be customized with additional Paleo-friendly ingredients such as diced tomatoes or a sprinkle of fresh herbs, elevating its taste profile while adhering to the principles of the Paleo diet.

These light and easy lunches are not only convenient but also prioritize nutritional balance. They are crafted to meet the demands of modern lifestyles, where time is often of the essence. Whether enjoyed at home or packed for work, these Paleo meals ensure that every bite contributes to sustained energy levels and overall well-being.

CHAPTER FIVE

DINNER RECIPES

Hearty Meat Dishes

This section delves into the world of satisfying, meat-centric dinners that form a core part of the Paleo diet. Emphasizing natural, unprocessed foods, the Paleo approach celebrates meat as a dietary staple. In this section, you'll discover a variety of recipes featuring beef, lamb, pork, and other meats, all designed to be both filling and nutritious. Each dish is thoughtfully crafted to incorporate vegetables and herbs, enhancing the natural flavors of the meat and providing a well-rounded, hearty meal.

Grilled Steak with Chimichurri Sauce

Imagine a juicy, perfectly grilled steak sizzling on your plate. This dish pairs the rich, savory flavor of the steak with a vibrant chimichurri sauce, made from fresh herbs, garlic, vinegar, and olive oil. The sauce adds a zesty, herbaceous touch that complements the meat beautifully. The result is a balanced dish that's both indulgent and wholesome, perfect for a Paleo dinner.

Slow-Cooked Pork Shoulder

Next, we have the slow-cooked pork shoulder. This recipe calls for tender, fall-apart pork shoulder that has been cooked slowly with a blend of spices and root vegetables. The slow cooking process allows the flavors to meld together, creating a dish that's rich and deeply satisfying. The pork becomes so tender that it almost melts in your mouth, while the vegetables add a subtle sweetness and earthiness to the meal. This dish is ideal for those who appreciate the comforting taste of slow-cooked meats and the convenience of a meal that can be prepared with minimal hands-on time.

Lamb Chops with Mint Pesto

For a slightly more exotic option, try the lamb chops with mint pesto. Lamb chops are already a luxurious choice, but when paired with a fresh, zesty mint pesto, they become truly exceptional. The pesto, made from fresh mint leaves, garlic, nuts, and olive oil, adds a bright, refreshing flavor that cuts through the richness of the lamb.

This dish is perfect for special occasions or when you want to treat yourself to something a bit different. The combination of the succulent lamb and the vibrant pesto is sure to impress and satisfy even the most discerning palate.

These recipes are perfect for those who love robust, meaty flavors and are looking for meals that will keep them full and satisfied. Each dish not only celebrates the essence of the Paleo diet but also showcases the versatility and depth of flavors that can be achieved with simple, wholesome ingredients. Whether you're a seasoned cook or just starting out, these hearty meat dishes are sure to become staples in your Paleo meal rotation, bringing warmth, comfort, and nutrition to your table.

Seafood And Fish Delights

Seafood and fish are nutritional powerhouses, offering a rich source of protein, omega-3 fatty acids, and essential nutrients, making them a staple in the Paleo diet. Seafood and Fish Delights, brings together an array of delectable recipes featuring a variety of fish such as salmon, tuna, and cod, along with shellfish like shrimp, scallops, and mussels. The focus of these recipes is to accentuate the natural flavors of the seafood, utilizing minimal seasoning and straightforward cooking methods to preserve their intrinsic taste and nutritional value.

One of the standout recipes is Baked Salmon with Lemon and Dill. This classic dish brings out the best in fresh salmon, a fish known for its rich flavor and high omega-3 content. The preparation is simple yet elegant: fresh salmon fillets are lightly seasoned with a drizzle of olive oil, a generous squeeze of lemon juice, and a sprinkle of dill. The fish is then baked to perfection, resulting in a moist and flavorful dish that is both healthy and satisfying. The combination of lemon and dill enhances the salmon's natural flavors, making this dish a go-to option for a quick and nutritious meal.

Another highlight is the Shrimp Stir-Fry. This recipe is perfect for busy weeknights, as it comes together quickly and effortlessly. It features succulent shrimp, which cook in a matter of minutes, paired with vibrant bell peppers that add a pop of color and crunch. The dish is finished with a savory garlic-ginger sauce, adding a depth of flavor that complements the shrimp perfectly. The result is a lively, nutritious stir-fry that is sure to become a family favorite. This recipe not only meets the dietary guidelines of the Paleo diet but also provides a delicious and visually appealing meal.

For those who enjoy the luxurious texture of shellfish, Seared Scallops with Garlic Butter is an absolute must-try. Scallops, known for their tender and slightly sweet flavor, are seared to golden-brown perfection. The key to achieving the perfect sear is to cook the scallops in a hot pan with a small amount of oil until they form a caramelized crust. They are then finished with a luscious garlic butter sauce, which adds a rich, savory dimension to the dish. The garlic butter not only enhances the natural sweetness of the scallops but also provides a mouthwatering finish that will impress any seafood lover.

Poultry Favorites

Poultry, including chicken and turkey, is a cornerstone of the Paleo diet, offering a rich source of lean protein that supports muscle growth, weight management, and overall health. This selection of recipes highlights the versatility and delicious potential of poultry, showcasing a variety of cooking methods and flavor profiles to suit any palate.

One standout dish is roasted chicken with herbs, a classic that never fails to impress. To prepare this, you need a whole chicken, seasoned generously with a blend of fresh herbs such as rosemary, thyme, and sage, along with minced garlic and slices of lemon. The combination of these ingredients not only infuses the chicken with a fragrant aroma but also keeps the meat tender and juicy. Roasting the chicken in the oven allows the skin to crisp up beautifully while the meat remains succulent, making it a perfect centerpiece for any meal.

For those who prefer a quicker, lighter option, grilled chicken breast with avocado salsa is an excellent choice. Start by marinating chicken breasts in olive oil, lime juice, and a touch of chili powder for a bit of heat. Grill the chicken until it's perfectly charred and cooked through. The real star of this dish, however, is the avocado salsa. Made with ripe avocados, diced tomatoes, red onion, cilantro, and a squeeze of lime juice, the salsa is fresh, creamy, and vibrant, providing a delightful contrast to the smoky grilled chicken. This dish is not only easy to prepare but also packed with nutrients, making it an ideal choice for a healthy, satisfying meal.

Another delicious option is turkey meatballs in tomato sauce, a comforting dish that brings warmth and flavor to the table. To make the meatballs, combine ground turkey with finely chopped onions, garlic, parsley, and a handful of almond flour to bind the mixture. Season with salt, pepper, and Italian herbs, then shape the mixture into small balls. Brown the meatballs in a skillet, then simmer them in a rich tomato sauce made from crushed tomatoes, garlic, onions, and a splash of balsamic vinegar for added depth. The result is tender, flavorful meatballs bathed in a luscious sauce, perfect for serving over a bed of zucchini noodles or alongside roasted vegetables.

These recipes demonstrate the adaptability of poultry in the Paleo diet, offering a variety of ways to enjoy this nutritious protein. Whether you're in the mood for a hearty roast, a light and fresh grilled dish, or a comforting bowl of meatballs, these options ensure that poultry remains a staple in your culinary repertoire, providing both nourishment and delight.

Vegetable-Centric Mains

While the Paleo diet often brings to mind images of meat-centric meals, vegetables hold an equally important place in this nutritional approach. Emphasizing the versatility and nutritional value of vegetables, this part of our culinary journey showcases main dishes where vegetables shine as the star ingredient. These recipes are not only hearty and satisfying but also demonstrate that vegetables can be just as filling and delicious as their meaty counterparts.

Take, for instance, stuffed bell peppers. These colorful vegetables are hollowed out and filled with a delectable mixture of ground meat, cauliflower rice, and assorted vegetables. The ground meat adds a savory richness, while the cauliflower rice offers a grain-free, nutrient-packed alternative to traditional rice. Combined with a medley of vegetables, this dish is a perfect example of how vegetables can create a satisfying and flavorful main course.

Another standout dish is eggplant lasagna. Instead of using traditional pasta, thin slices of roasted eggplant are layered with a rich marinara sauce and a creamy, cashew-based "cheese" sauce. This innovative take on lasagna retains the comfort and heartiness of the classic dish while aligning with Paleo principles. The roasted eggplant provides a robust, slightly smoky flavor that pairs beautifully with the tangy marinara and the velvety cashew "cheese," making it a delightful and nutritious meal.

For a lighter, yet equally satisfying option, zucchini noodles with pesto are a fantastic choice. Spiralized zucchini, often referred to as "zoodles," serve as a fresh, low-carb substitute for traditional pasta. Tossed with a vibrant, homemade pesto sauce, these noodles offer a burst of flavor and a refreshing crunch. The pesto, made from fresh basil, garlic, pine nuts, and olive oil, adds a zesty and aromatic quality that complements the zucchini perfectly. This dish highlights how vegetables can be transformed into creative and mouthwatering meals.

These vegetable-centric mains are designed to celebrate the diversity and nutritional benefits of vegetables within the Paleo framework. Each recipe showcases how vegetables can take center stage, providing not only a variety of flavors and textures but also essential vitamins and minerals. By incorporating these dishes into your meal plan, you can enjoy the full spectrum of what the Paleo diet has to offer, all while relishing the delightful and satisfying nature of vegetable-based cuisine. These recipes prove that with a bit of creativity, vegetables can be the hero of your plate, delivering both taste and nourishment in every bite.

One-Pot And Sheet Pan Dinners

For those who prefer minimal cleanup and easy preparation, this section offers a selection of recipes that can be made in a single pot or on a sheet pan. These dishes are designed to be simple, convenient, and packed with flavor, making them perfect for busy weeknights or when you simply want a hassle-free cooking experience.

One such recipe is Sheet Pan Chicken and Vegetables. This dish brings together juicy chicken thighs and a colorful array of vegetables, all roasted to perfection on a single sheet pan. The beauty of this recipe lies in its simplicity: you can use whatever vegetables you have on hand, making it a great way to clean out your fridge.

Common choices include bell peppers, zucchini, and red onions, all tossed with olive oil, salt, pepper, and your favorite herbs. The chicken and vegetables cook together, allowing the flavors to meld and creating a deliciously satisfying meal with minimal effort and cleanup.

Another fantastic one-pot option is Beef Stew. This comforting classic is made with tender chunks of beef, hearty root vegetables like carrots and potatoes, and a rich, savory broth. Everything is cooked together in one pot, allowing the flavors to develop and deepen as the stew simmers. The result is a warm, nourishing dish that's perfect for a cozy night in. The best part? You can let it cook slowly on the stovetop or in a slow cooker, giving you plenty of hands-off time to relax or take care of other tasks.

CHAPTER SIX

SNACKS AND SIDES

Paleo-Friendly Snacks

The Paleo diet promotes consuming whole, unprocessed foods that mirror those eaten by our hunter-gatherer ancestors. This dietary approach emphasizes natural, nutrient-dense options, making snacking a healthy and satisfying experience. Paleo-friendly snacks are an essential component of this diet, providing nourishment and energy without compromising on the principles of clean eating.

Fruits, vegetables, nuts, and seeds are the cornerstones of Paleo snacking. Fresh fruits, such as apples, berries, and oranges, are excellent choices. Apples offer a satisfying crunch and are rich in fiber, which aids digestion and helps maintain stable blood sugar levels. Berries, like strawberries, blueberries, and raspberries, are not only delicious but also packed with antioxidants, vitamins, and minerals. Oranges, with their natural sweetness, provide a quick energy boost and a hefty dose of vitamin C, which is crucial for immune health.

Vegetables are another fantastic snack option. Carrot sticks, cucumber slices, and bell pepper strips are not only easy to prepare but also brimming with vitamins and minerals. Carrots, for instance, are high in beta-carotene, which the body converts to vitamin A, essential for vision and immune function. Cucumbers are incredibly hydrating, making them a refreshing snack, especially in warmer weather. Bell peppers are rich in vitamins

A and C, adding a nutritional punch to your snack plate.

Pairing fruits and vegetables with a small portion of nuts or seeds can elevate your snack by adding healthy fats and protein. Almonds, walnuts, and pumpkin seeds are all Paleo-approved and can help keep you full between meals. Almonds are a great source of vitamin E and magnesium, while walnuts provide omega-3 fatty acids, which support heart health. Pumpkin seeds, or pepitas, are rich in zinc and iron, essential for immune function and energy production.

For those who prefer more substantial snacks, homemade energy bars or balls can be an excellent choice. These can be made using dates, nuts, and a bit of coconut oil. Dates provide natural sweetness and are high in fiber and potassium, which are vital for maintaining healthy blood pressure and muscle function. Nuts add crunch and protein, making the snack more satisfying. Coconut oil not only helps bind the ingredients together but also adds a dose of medium-chain triglycerides (MCTs), which can provide a quick source of energy.

Nut And Seed Treats

Nuts and seeds are essential components of the Paleo diet, prized for their rich nutrient profiles and healthy fats. These versatile ingredients can be enjoyed on their own or transformed into delightful treats that align perfectly with the Paleo philosophy.

Among the most popular choices are almonds, walnuts, and cashews, which can be easily prepared by roasting to enhance their natural flavors and provide a satisfying crunch. Perfect for quick snacking, these roasted nuts can also be stored conveniently for whenever cravings strike. For those with a sweet tooth, nut clusters offer a delightful option. Simply combine your preferred nuts with a touch of natural sweetness from honey or maple syrup, then bake until they achieve a delectable crispness.

Seeds such as chia, flax, and sunflower seeds are equally versatile in Paleo cooking. Chia seeds, for instance, can be transformed into a creamy pudding by soaking them in almond milk infused with vanilla and a hint of honey. This nutritious snack not only satisfies cravings but also provides a boost of omega-3 fatty acids and fiber. Meanwhile, roasted pumpkin seeds seasoned with aromatic spices offer a savory alternative, delivering a crunchy texture and a wealth of nutrients in every bite.

The appeal of nuts and seeds in Paleo cuisine extends beyond snacking. They serve as foundational ingredients in various recipes, adding depth and nutritional value to dishes ranging from salads to baked goods. Their versatility allows them to be incorporated into breakfast options like homemade granola or sprinkled over fruit salads for added texture and flavor.

Savory Sides And Veggies

Vegetables are not just a side dish in the Paleo diet; they are a cornerstone, providing essential nutrients like vitamins, minerals, and fiber. Incorporating savory sides and veggie dishes into your meals not only enhances nutritional intake but also adds delightful flavors and textures.

Roasted Vegetables: One of the simplest and most flavorful ways to prepare vegetables in the Paleo diet is roasting. Take vegetables like sweet potatoes, Brussels sprouts, and cauliflower, cut them into bite-sized pieces, toss them in olive oil, and season generously with herbs and spices like rosemary, thyme, or paprika. Roast in the oven until they're tender and caramelized. This method intensifies their natural sweetness and brings out a delicious depth of flavor.

Vegetable Chips: For a crunchy snack or a creative side dish, consider making vegetable chips. Thinly slice root vegetables such as beets, carrots, or parsnips using a mandoline slicer or a sharp knife. Toss them lightly in olive oil, sprinkle with sea salt or your favorite seasoning blend, and bake until crispy. These homemade chips are not only satisfyingly crunchy but also packed with nutrients, offering a healthier alternative to store-bought potato chips.

Veggie Stir-Fry: Stir-frying is another fantastic technique for preparing vegetables while retaining their crispness and vibrant colors. Heat coconut oil in a pan and add a mix of your favorite vegetables, such as bell peppers, broccoli, snap peas, and mushrooms. Season with minced garlic, grated ginger, and a splash of tamari sauce or coconut aminos for umami richness. Stir-fry until the vegetables are just tender-crisp, preserving their nutritional value and natural flavors.

Incorporating Variety: The key to enjoying vegetables on the Paleo diet is variety. Experiment with different combinations and cooking methods to keep meals exciting and satisfying. Consider adding roasted asparagus with lemon zest, sautéed spinach with garlic and pine nuts, or a colorful salad of mixed greens with avocado and cherry tomatoes.

Dips And Sauces

Dips and sauces are essential components of a Paleo diet, adding depth and flavor to snacks and meals while staying true to nutritional principles. One of the most beloved Paleo dips is guacamole, a creamy blend of ripe avocados, lime juice, and a touch of salt. Its rich texture and healthy fats make it an ideal companion for veggie sticks or homemade tortilla chips.

Guacamole not only satisfies cravings but also provides essential nutrients like potassium and fiber, essential for a balanced diet.

Another staple is salsa, vibrant and fresh with diced tomatoes, onions, cilantro, and a splash of lime juice. This zesty combination not only enhances the taste of dishes but also contributes vitamins A and C from tomatoes, along with antioxidants from cilantro. It's a versatile option that pairs well with grilled meats or simply as a dip for crunchy snacks.

For those seeking a unique twist, Paleo-friendly hummus offers a satisfying alternative to traditional chickpea-based varieties. By substituting roasted cauliflower or zucchini for chickpeas and blending them with tahini, lemon juice, and garlic, you get a creamy, flavorful dip. This variation retains the creamy texture and nutty flavor profile of classic hummus while adding a dose of dietary fiber and vitamins from the vegetables.

Pesto, traditionally made with fresh basil, pine nuts, and olive oil, is another Paleo-friendly sauce that complements various dishes. It serves as both a dip and a sauce, enriching roasted vegetables or grilled meats with its aromatic basil and nutty undertones. Pesto provides healthy monounsaturated fats from olive oil and pine nuts, promoting heart health and satiety.

These Paleo dips and sauces aren't just about flavor; they're nutritional powerhouses. Avocados in guacamole offer healthy monounsaturated fats, while tomatoes in salsa provide vitamins and antioxidants. The roasted vegetables in Paleo hummus contribute fiber and essential minerals, and pesto's basil and olive oil combination delivers anti-inflammatory properties and supports immune function.

Incorporating these dips and sauces into a Paleo diet not only enhances taste but also ensures a balanced intake of essential nutrients. Whether enjoyed as a snack with raw vegetables or as a sauce drizzled over a hearty meal, these options cater to both culinary enjoyment and nutritional well-being. By embracing these Paleo-friendly choices, individuals can savor delicious flavors while promoting overall health and vitality.

Energy Boosting Bites

Energy-boosting snacks provide a quick pick-me-up whenever you need a burst of vitality. These snacks are meticulously crafted to deliver sustained energy through a blend of healthy fats, proteins, and natural sugars. One of the most favored options is energy balls, created by blending dates, nuts, and a hint of coconut oil into a cohesive dough, which is then rolled into convenient, bite-sized spheres. These versatile treats can be enriched with flavors such as cocoa powder, vanilla extract, or a sprinkle of cinnamon to suit various tastes.

Another popular choice is trail mix, a harmonious medley of nuts, seeds, and dried fruits like raisins or cranberries. This combination not only satisfies cravings but also offers a nutrient-packed punch ideal for active lifestyles. For those craving a more indulgent option, consider whipping up Paleo-friendly fudge. This delectable treat involves mixing coconut oil, cocoa powder, and a touch of honey, then chilling until firm. The result is a rich, satisfying confection that aligns with Paleo dietary principles while providing a guilt-free indulgence.

Energy bites are not just nutritious; they're also incredibly convenient for on-the-go snacking, fitting perfectly into busy schedules and demanding routines. Whether you're heading to the gym, embarking on a hike, or simply need a mid-afternoon boost at work, these snacks offer a delicious solution. They're designed to sustain energy levels without the crash associated with sugary snacks or processed foods, making them an excellent choice for those seeking balanced nutrition.

By incorporating wholesome ingredients like nuts, seeds, and natural sweeteners, these snacks not only support energy levels but also contribute to overall well-being. The combination of healthy fats and proteins helps stabilize blood sugar levels, promoting sustained energy release throughout the day. Moreover, the natural sugars from dates or dried fruits provide a quick source of energy, ideal for replenishing glycogen stores after exercise or during moments of fatigue.

CHAPTER SEVEN

DESSERTS AND TREATS

Paleo Baking Basics

Paleo baking represents a culinary approach that eschews traditional wheat flour in favor of nutrient-dense alternatives, catering to those following the Paleo diet. Central to this baking philosophy are alternative flours such as almond flour, coconut flour, and tapioca flour. These substitutes not only impart unique textures but also enrich baked goods with a spectrum of vitamins, minerals, and healthy fats absent in conventional wheat flour.

Almond flour, derived from finely ground almonds, stands out for its rich flavor and moist texture. It serves as a versatile base for various recipes, including cakes, cookies, and muffins, offering a gluten-free option that aligns with Paleo principles. Coconut flour, another prominent choice, derives from dried coconut meat finely ground into a powdery consistency. This flour is highly absorbent, requiring more liquid in recipes, but it contributes a subtly sweet taste and a soft, moist crumb to baked treats.

Tapioca flour, extracted from cassava root, rounds out the trio of Paleo-friendly flours. It provides a light, airy texture to baked goods and serves as an excellent thickener for sauces and soups due to its neutral taste and gluten-free nature. Together, these alternative flours allow Paleo enthusiasts to enjoy a wide array of baked goods without compromising their dietary preferences.

In Paleo baking, sweeteners play a crucial role in enhancing flavor while maintaining a low glycemic index. Natural options such as honey, maple syrup, and coconut sugar are preferred over refined sugars. Honey, a time-honored sweetener, offers not only sweetness but also trace amounts of essential nutrients and antioxidants. Maple syrup, derived from the sap of maple trees, imparts a distinctive flavor profile, making it a popular choice for pancakes, muffins, and glazes. Coconut sugar, made from the sap of coconut palm trees, provides a caramel-like sweetness with a lower glycemic index than regular sugar, making it a suitable alternative for those mindful of blood sugar levels.

These natural sweeteners are used sparingly in Paleo baking, aligning with the diet's emphasis on whole, unprocessed foods. They not only add sweetness but also contribute subtle nuances to baked goods, enhancing their overall flavor profile without the need for artificial additives or excessive refined sugars.

Fruit-Based Desserts

In the realm of Paleo desserts, fruits emerge as vibrant protagonists, wielding natural sweetness alongside a bounty of essential vitamins and antioxidants. These desserts celebrate the simplicity and goodness of fresh produce, offering not just indulgence but also healthful nourishment.

Imagine a dessert tableau where fresh berries glisten under a veil of velvety coconut cream, their tangy sweetness harmonizing with the rich, tropical undertones of coconut. Each bite is a revelation, a burst of flavors that transports you to sun-dappled orchards and verdant berry patches. This combination not only satiates cravings for sweetness but also fortifies your body with fiber and a spectrum of vital nutrients.

Then there are the grilled peaches, their tender flesh kissed by flames until golden and aromatic. A delicate drizzle of honey, warmed by the grill's touch, cascades over each slice, enhancing the peach's natural sugars without veering from Paleo principles. This dessert embodies the art of simplicity—minimal ingredients, maximum flavor—capturing the essence of seasonal abundance in every bite.

For those seeking a lighter yet equally delightful option, a refreshing fruit salad beckons. Here, the medley of seasonal fruits—crisp apples, succulent grapes, perhaps a hint of citrus—unites in a symphony of colors and textures. Dressed lightly with a squeeze of fresh lemon juice or a sprinkle of mint leaves, this salad is a testament to the Paleo philosophy of embracing whole, unprocessed foods. Each spoonful offers not just sweetness but also a refreshing crunch and a burst of hydration, making it an ideal conclusion to any meal.

These fruit-centric desserts go beyond mere culinary indulgence; they embody the Paleo commitment to nourishment through natural ingredients. They invite you to savor the bounty of nature, offering a guilt-free way to satisfy your sweet tooth while honoring your body's need for wholesome nutrition. Whether enjoyed alone or shared among friends, these desserts enrich your Paleo journey, reminding you that eating well can be both a pleasure and a celebration of health.

Decadent Chocolate Treats

Indulging in chocolate while on the Paleo diet doesn't have to be a guilty pleasure. Embracing the philosophy of clean eating doesn't mean sacrificing the rich, decadent taste of chocolate. For enthusiasts of this ancient diet, dark chocolate emerges as a delightful exception—a treat that fits within the framework of Paleo principles.

The key to enjoying chocolate on the Paleo diet lies in choosing varieties with a high cocoa content, ideally 70% or higher. This selection ensures minimal processing and a concentration of cocoa solids, imparting a robust flavor without the excessive sugars found in conventional chocolate bars. Dark chocolate not only satisfies cravings but also delivers a generous dose of antioxidants, compounds known for their health-boosting properties.

There are numerous ways to savor dark chocolate on a Paleo regime. A straightforward approach involves relishing small pieces of high-quality dark chocolate on its own, allowing its deep, bittersweet notes to unfold slowly. For those inclined towards culinary adventures, integrating dark chocolate into Paleo-friendly recipes opens up a realm of creative possibilities.

Imagine crafting velvety chocolate truffles, where the intense cocoa flavor harmonizes with coconut cream and a hint of vanilla essence. These truffles, rolled delicately in cocoa powder or shredded coconut, provide a luxurious treat that's both satisfying and nutritionally balanced.

Alternatively, delve into the realm of desserts with a Paleo twist. Indulge in a luscious chocolate mousse enriched with ripe avocados and cocoa, blending until silky smooth. This creamy delight offers a guilt-free alternative to traditional dairy-laden desserts, combining the richness of chocolate with the wholesome goodness of avocados.

For those seeking a textural contrast, consider preparing a decadent chocolate bark adorned with a sprinkle of nuts and dried fruits. Dark chocolate, melted and spread thinly, becomes the canvas for a mosaic of flavors and textures—crunchy almonds, tart cranberries, or the natural sweetness of dried apricots—all coming together in a symphony of taste and nutrition.

Each of these creations exemplifies the versatility of dark chocolate within the Paleo diet. By choosing high-quality ingredients and embracing natural sweetness from fruits and nuts, these treats not only satisfy cravings but also align with the principles of clean eating. They represent a celebration of flavor, texture, and mindful indulgence—a testament to how ancient wisdom can harmonize with modern culinary creativity.

Grain-Free Cookies And Bars

Grain-free cookies and bars stand as quintessential elements within the realm of Paleo dessert recipes. These delectable treats, crafted from almond flour or coconut flour, offer a wholesome alternative to their grain-laden counterparts. Embracing the core principles of Paleo, they eschew grains and instead harness the nutritive power of nut-based flours, alongside enriching ingredients like nut butters, eggs, and natural sweeteners.

Almond flour and coconut flour emerge as foundational components, lending a distinct texture and flavor profile to each creation. Almond flour, renowned for its fine consistency and mild nutty taste, forms a robust base that holds together well in baking. Meanwhile, coconut flour, derived from dried coconut meat, imbues treats with a subtly sweet essence and a delightful lightness.

The amalgamation of these flours with nut butters such as almond or cashew introduces a rich, creamy element, enhancing both taste and nutritional value. Eggs play a crucial role, binding the ingredients while contributing protein and structure. Natural sweeteners like honey, maple syrup, or coconut sugar offer a gentle sweetness that complements the earthy tones of the flours, ensuring each bite satisfies the palate without compromising on healthfulness.

To elevate these creations, artisans of Paleo baking often incorporate enticing additions. Dark chocolate chips, renowned for their antioxidant properties and indulgent taste, add bursts of richness. Nuts such as pecans, walnuts, or almonds contribute a satisfying crunch and additional nutrients, while dried fruits like cranberries or apricots infuse bursts of natural sweetness and chewiness.

In crafting grain-free cookies and bars, adherence to Paleo principles extends beyond mere exclusion of grains; it embraces a holistic approach to ingredients that nourish and delight. Each batch represents a harmonious blend of flavors and textures, offering a guilt-free indulgence that satisfies cravings without straying from a health-conscious lifestyle.

Special Occasion Desserts

Special occasions call for desserts that not only delight the taste buds but also align with the principles of the Paleo diet, showcasing creativity and wholesome ingredients. Paleo desserts, designed to impress even the most discerning guests, elevate traditional treats into nutritious indulgences that everyone can enjoy guilt-free.

Imagine a Paleo cheesecake, crafted from creamy cashews and coconut cream, adorned with a vibrant array of fresh berries. This decadent creation not only satisfies sweet cravings but also delivers a rich, velvety texture that rivals conventional cheesecakes. Each bite is a testament to the artistry of Paleo baking, where natural ingredients harmonize to create a dessert that's as nourishing as it is delicious.

For those who prefer a warm, comforting dessert, a Paleo-friendly apple crisp offers a delightful alternative. Picture juicy apples, sliced and baked to tender perfection, crowned with a crumbly topping made from nuts and coconut flour. The combination of sweet fruit and nutty crunch embodies the essence of Paleo cuisine, providing a satisfying end to any celebratory meal.

What sets these desserts apart is their ability to cater to dietary preferences without compromising on flavor or presentation. Whether it's a birthday, anniversary, or holiday gathering, Paleo desserts prove that indulgence can coexist with nutritional mindfulness. They demonstrate that wholesome ingredients like nuts, fruits, and coconut products can be transformed into culinary masterpieces that captivate both palate and imagination.

Moreover, the versatility of Paleo baking allows for endless creativity. From intricate decorations to personalized flavors, Paleo dessert makers can tailor each creation to match the theme and atmosphere of the occasion. This adaptability ensures that every dessert served is not only a treat for the senses but also a reflection of the care and thoughtfulness put into its preparation.

CHAPTER EIGHT

BEVERAGES

Paleo Smoothies And Juices

Smoothies and juices offer a refreshing and nutritious way to embrace the Paleo diet, focusing on whole, unprocessed ingredients that fuel your body with essential nutrients. When crafting smoothies and juices within the Paleo framework, the emphasis lies on using fresh, natural components such as leafy greens, fruits, and healthy fats like avocado or coconut milk. These choices not only enhance flavor but also contribute to a balanced intake of vitamins, minerals, and antioxidants, supporting overall health.

In the realm of smoothies, berries often take center stage due to their antioxidant properties and natural sweetness.

Combining berries with nutrient-rich leafy greens such as spinach or kale creates vibrant concoctions bursting with flavor and vitality. The addition of a creamy texture can be achieved by incorporating avocado or coconut milk, both of which provide healthy fats crucial for sustaining energy levels throughout the day.

Juices under the Paleo diet philosophy are similarly geared towards simplicity and wholesomeness. Citrus fruits like oranges or grapefruits lend a zesty tang while contributing a dose of vitamin C. Adding a hint of ginger not only enhances flavor but also brings its anti-inflammatory benefits to the mix. It's essential to refrain from processed sugars, instead opting for natural sweeteners in moderation, such as dates or honey, to maintain the integrity of the Paleo principles.

Experimentation is key when exploring Paleo smoothies and juices. Blend different combinations to find your preferred balance of flavors and textures. For example, a tropical blend of pineapple, mango, and coconut milk transports you to an island getaway while nourishing your body with essential nutrients. Alternatively, a green smoothie featuring spinach, cucumber, and a touch of lemon offers a refreshing way to boost your daily intake of greens.

Herbal Teas And Infusions

Herbal teas offer a delightful and health-conscious way to hydrate while reaping numerous benefits aligned with the Paleo diet philosophy. These natural infusions not only quench thirst but also provide soothing effects and health boosts without the additives and artificial flavors found in many commercial beverages.

Paleo enthusiasts favor herbal teas for their purity and diverse health benefits. Chamomile, renowned for its calming properties, stands out as a favorite choice among tea drinkers seeking relaxation and stress relief. Its gentle floral aroma and mild, slightly sweet taste make it perfect for winding down after a long day or preparing for a restful night's sleep.

Peppermint tea is another popular option within the Paleo community, valued for its digestive benefits. Its refreshing, minty flavor not only aids digestion but also helps alleviate bloating and discomfort, making it an ideal choice after meals or whenever a digestive pick-me-up is needed.

Rooibos tea, derived from the leaves of the South African red bush plant, boasts a rich profile of antioxidants. Paleo followers appreciate its earthy, slightly sweet flavor and its potential to support overall health and well-being. Rooibos is particularly noted for its anti-inflammatory properties and its ability to promote skin health, making it a versatile addition to any Paleo tea collection.

When preparing herbal teas, Paleo enthusiasts emphasize the importance of using high-quality ingredients free from additives and artificial enhancements. Whether enjoyed hot on a chilly day or chilled over ice during warmer months, these teas can be personalized with a slice of lemon or a touch of raw honey for added flavor, aligning perfectly with the Paleo preference for natural, unprocessed foods.

Paleo Coffee Alternatives

In the realm of Paleo dietary practices, coffee alternatives abound for enthusiasts seeking to sidestep the acidity and potential crash associated with traditional coffee consumption. These alternatives not only cater to diverse tastes but also align with the principles of Paleo, emphasizing natural, nutrient-dense options.

One prominent substitute gaining popularity among Paleo adherents is roasted dandelion root tea. Renowned for its robust flavor reminiscent of coffee, this herbal brew offers a satisfying alternative without the jolt of caffeine. It's appreciated not just for its taste but also for its potential health benefits, including support for liver function and digestion.

For those craving a creamy texture akin to traditional lattes without dairy, Paleo-friendly options like coconut milk or almond milk lattes step in admirably. These plant-based alternatives not only enhance the richness of the beverage but also contribute beneficial fats and a touch of natural sweetness. They serve as versatile bases that can be customized with spices such as cinnamon or nutmeg, enhancing both flavor and nutritional value.

Another stalwart in the world of Paleo coffee substitutes is matcha green tea. Renowned for its vibrant green hue and distinctive flavor, matcha provides a sustained energy boost attributed to its moderate caffeine content, which is less likely to induce the sharp peaks and crashes associated with coffee. Beyond its energizing properties, matcha is celebrated for its high antioxidant levels, promoting overall health and well-being.

For those exploring Paleo dietary principles, these coffee alternatives not only offer variety but also align with the philosophy of consuming whole, unprocessed foods. Whether it's the earthy notes of roasted dandelion root tea, the creamy indulgence of coconut or almond milk lattes, or the invigorating properties of matcha green tea, each option presents a pathway to enjoying a satisfying beverage without compromising on health goals.

Hydrating Drinks And Electrolyte Boosters

Staying properly hydrated is crucial when following the Paleo diet, particularly if you maintain an active lifestyle. Hydration not only supports overall health but also aids in maintaining energy levels and supporting bodily functions.

One excellent natural option for replenishing electrolytes on the Paleo diet is coconut water. It's prized for its rich content of potassium and magnesium, essential minerals that play key roles in muscle function, hydration, and overall well-being. Unlike many commercial sports drinks that often contain added sugars and artificial ingredients, coconut water offers a clean, natural source of hydration. It's particularly beneficial after physical activity, helping to restore electrolyte balance and prevent dehydration.

To create your own homemade electrolyte drink, start with fresh coconut water. Look for varieties that are pure and free from added sugars or artificial flavors to maintain the Paleo-friendly aspect. Coconut water already contains potassium, magnesium, and sodium, which are crucial electrolytes lost through sweat during exercise. Adding a pinch of sea salt further enhances the electrolyte profile of your drink, aiding in rehydration. Sea salt provides sodium, another essential electrolyte that helps maintain fluid balance and supports nerve and muscle function.

For a refreshing twist, include a splash of freshly squeezed lemon juice in your homemade electrolyte drink. Lemon juice not only adds a burst of flavor but also provides a natural source of vitamin C, which can help support immune function and provide antioxidant benefits. The combination of coconut water, sea salt, and lemon juice creates a hydrating beverage that is both refreshing and beneficial for replenishing electrolytes lost during physical exertion.

When preparing your electrolyte drink, ensure all ingredients are well mixed to distribute the electrolytes evenly throughout the beverage. You can adjust the flavor by adding more or less lemon juice according to your taste preferences. This homemade option not only supports your Paleo diet goals but also allows you to customize your hydration strategy based on your activity level and personal preferences.

Festive Paleo Cocktails And Mocktails

Even within the Paleo framework, celebrations can still be vibrant and enjoyable. For those adhering strictly to Paleo principles or simply looking to avoid alcohol, mocktails offer a delightful alternative. These refreshing beverages are crafted using fresh fruit juices, sparkling water, and aromatic herbs such as basil or mint, lending a burst of natural flavors without straying from Paleo guidelines.

Mocktails are perfect for any occasion, offering a guilt-free way to indulge in festive drinks. Imagine sipping on a cool Watermelon Mint Cooler, where freshly blended watermelon juice meets a hint of mint over ice, creating a symphony of summer flavors. Alternatively, a Sparkling Citrus Spritzer combines tangy citrus juices with fizzy sparkling water, garnished with a twist of lemon or lime, delivering a zesty sensation that tingles the taste buds.

For those who occasionally partake in alcohol, Paleo-friendly cocktails can still be enjoyed responsibly. Opt for spirits like tequila or vodka, which are lower in sugar and gluten-free, ensuring they align with Paleo dietary guidelines. Pair these spirits with natural mixers such as freshly squeezed lime juice or coconut water for a tropical twist. The result? Cocktails like a refreshing Tequila Sunrise, where tequila meets fresh orange juice and a hint of grenadine, offering a balance of sweetness and tanginess in each sip.

It's important to approach alcoholic beverages with moderation and prioritize hydration. For those choosing mocktails, the abundance of hydrating ingredients ensures that each sip not only satisfies but also contributes to your overall well-being. Whether you're celebrating a special occasion or simply winding down after a long day, these Paleo cocktails and mocktails provide a flavorful way to stay true to your dietary choices without compromising on taste or enjoyment.

THE END